Prostate Cancer Let's Talk!
Written and narrated by – Edgar Lloyd

Prostate Cancer

Let's Talk!

ISBN: 9798488053861

Copyright © 2021 by Edgar Lloyd
All rights reserved. In accordance with the U.S. Copyright Act of 1976, the scanning, uploading, and electronic sharing of any part of this book without permission of the Author/Publisher is unlawful piracy and theft of the author's intellectual property.

Dedication

I would like to dedicate this book to my wife, Dawn, my daughter, Amber, and my son-in-law, Rocky. They have provided me with the strength to ride out this wave of uncertainty. You will never know how much you all mean to me...Bless you guys.

I would be remiss if I didn't mention my mother, as she has graciously provided her heart, love, and insight in helping me stay the course. She is a survivor, and her strength is truly an inspiration.
Stay Blessed.

To my best friends Ray Valadez, and Roy Valadez, for their vigilance in metaphorically wrapping their arms around me. Their prayers, and the prayers of the amassed "prayer army" they've assembled on my behalf, have helped me greatly in bearing this burden...Bless you all.

Special thanks to Pastor, Dr. Daniel C. Okpara (Shining Light Christian Centre) for his friendship and prayers during this most trying of times. He has been an inspiration to me both, as an author, and as a Christian leader in his country.

Special thanks to my avid cyclist friend, and fellow musician, Don Caravella, for his friendship and willingness to share his experiences with me concerning this dreaded monster. He's a survivor, and will be in my life for as long as I am here...Bless you, my friend.

Shout out to JPS Hospital in FT. Worth, TX. for the kind and professional manner in which they conduct business. Truly a first-class facility.

Finally, to all the friends, family, and other survivors who have reached out to me with their concern. It has truly been a humbling experience. I wish you all great health, prosperity, and happiness...
My most heartfelt Blessings go out to each and every one of you.

CONTENTS

Contents

Introduction i
Chapter 1 - My First Doctors Visit - The GP v
Chapter 2 – Insurance 1
Chapter 3 - The Urologist 9
Chapter 5 – The Biopsy 15
Chapter 6 – The Results 19
Chapter 7 - The Scans 23
Chapter 8 - Scan 2 – Not Like The First. 27
Chapter 9 – The Surgeon's Consult 33
Chapter 10 – The MRI Experience – Well, I Tried 41
Chapter 11 – The MRI – Round 2 47
Chapter 12 - The MRI Results 57
Chapter 13 - The Surgery 61
Thoughts From The Author 69
About The Author 71

Introduction

"I will say of the Lord, He is my refuge and my fortress, my God, in whom I trust."

(Psalm 91:2)

Ok, I'm turning 67 in a few weeks, February 16th, 2021, and I have not been to a doctor's office in 40+ years. Not bragging about that, because in retrospect it was a stupid decision, but I had never really felt a reason to go. I've only been sick (Cold or Flu, etc.) a few days in my life, and although slightly overweight (about 30 lbs.) I feel great. I guess you could say that, to some degree, my male ego has played a part, although I've never had that macho thing of being *"strong like bull,"* my reticence, or stubbornness, mainly stemmed from the fact that I've never had health insurance. That has always been the major factor in my decisions not to go for checkups. I'm self-employed, make a modest income, and although I'm not broke mind you, I've never had much disposable income, and health insurance seemed like a luxury. I just reasoned, that I could always go to the county hospital if something major happened. As true as that is, regular doctor's visits, and the like, do cost money.

Back when I reached 50, the seemingly "magic" age for an overall checkup, I toyed with the idea of getting a physical, but I missed that one. I just figured at some point in the future I would go. Well, it took 17 years for that day to show up. Again, not smart.

So, how did I get to this point? Just prior to my 67th birthday, my daughter, Amber, and wife, Dawn insisted that I make an appointment to see a doctor to at least get a once over. A week went by, and I hadn't made an appointment. That's when they walked into my studio with an appointment slip. On their own, they had made an appointment for me to see a doctor.

I marked the day of my appointment on my calendar, and although, I felt good overall, I was having bathroom issues, so I felt good about seeing a doctor. I didn't have any pain, or anything to cause alarm, but the frequency of bathroom trips throughout the night had increased, averaging six, or more, times. Fully emptying my bladder, had also become a concern, as my stream, or flow, had become intermittent. I knew I wasn't finished, so I would squeeze myself in order to create some back pressure, in order to release another stream. I would find myself doing that, 3 or 4 times, before I felt I was finished urinating. Then, there were times that I could barely get to the bathroom in time. My house is not that big, and no matter where I was in my house, this little inconvenience should not have been a concern, but it was, so I gave in to the fact that it was probably a good idea to see a doctor.

Until this bathroom concern appeared, I had never really paid attention to the plethora of TV commercials relating to this issue, I now found myself tuned into them, and was willing to give some over the counter remedies a try. I tried several, like Saw palmetto etc., but nothing really worked, so I went to the internet to do some research. This is not usually a good idea, as the glut of information can overwhelm you, and can really play on your head. I did come away with this little tid-bit, however. Unless you get something from the doctor in the way of a prescription, the OTC (Over The Counter) stuff isn't very effective. So, don't waste your money. The problem is deeper than that.

Benign prostatic hyperplasia, or (BPH), is a real health issue that "all" men, let me repeat that, "all" men, at some point will have to face, to at least some degree. The numbers are staggering, and the older you get, the more likely you'll be faced with this problem. Let's hope we all see a 100, and going to the bathroom is our greatest issue.

Prayer

Heavenly Father, I speak to you today with the conviction that you are with me, that you will strengthen me, and help steer me through these trying times. You will uphold me with Your righteous right hand… in Jesus' name - Amen

Chapter 1 - My First Doctors Visit - The GP

"For in the day of trouble he will keep me safe in his dwelling; he will hide me in the shelter of his sacred tent and set me high upon a rock." - (Psalm 27:5 NIV)

My first doctor's visit, on March 5th, 2021, was nerve racking, as I was not used to being in a doctor's office, but I sat patiently, excuse the one of many puns to come, and eventually the doctor showed up. He was very kind, and quickly put me at ease. We talked about why I had decided to finally see a doctor, and I told him of my bathroom issues, and that I was specifically concerned about my Prostate. I knew that I should have gotten screened years ago, and was hoping I hadn't let any issues compound.

He expressed his approval of me starting to take an active role in my health, and then, very matter-of-factly, and out of the blue, asked me to lower my pants, and lay face down on the table. He suggested that I lean on my elbows, as that would make what was about to happen, and you and I both know what that is, a little easier on me. I complied, and he proceeded to insert his gloved and greased finger into my anus. There was no pain, just a little discomfort. I definitely knew he was there however, and I could feel him probing around, but it wasn't painful. He was there for about 10 seconds, and that was it. The exam was over.

"You can pull you pants up now." He directed.

I sat on the stool next to him, and he informed me that he had found a small growth on the left side of my Prostate that could be Cancerous, but a digital rectal exam, on its own, isn't the most definitive way to deduce if a growth is Cancerous. He suggested that I make an appointment with a Urologist, as soon as possible.

My first thoughts were, *'Cancer? Me? Really?'* That prospect hadn't entered my naive mind to this point, I was thinking I simply had a Prostate issue, but Cancer? That was a blow.

Prayer

Lord, I avow that I believe Your Word, and declare that You will never leave me, nor forsake me, that You are always with me, even in times that I feel lost, broken, and fearful. Even when I am overwhelmed by the situations I am in, I declare your presence…in Jesus' name – Amen

Chapter 2 – Insurance

"I will prosper and be in good health, even as my soul is flourishing, for my prosperity is God's will." – (3 John 1:2)

A month had gone by since my first doctors visit, which was in March, 2021, and the bill had arrived, it was a little over $200. Not huge, but I felt it was a harbinger of things to come, as I knew I had to see other doctors.

In the interim period, both my wife and daughter worked on acquiring health insurance for myself, and my wife, since she had lost her insurance after her lay off during the Covid onslaught. They found out that, surprisingly, if you do some research, you can get health insurance at a pretty reasonable rate. Depending on your income, you can get insurance for as little as free. Yup! Free! This depends on your income however, as these "marketplace" health companies, as they are called, use your income as a basis for premiums. If you do some homework, you can find the right company that best suits your financial situation. They're out there, so google the topic.

During 2020, my wife, after her lay off, was receiving workers compensation, and my job situation had pretty much dried up as well. As a result, we fit most of the qualifications to receive a reduced monthly premium, and we found a company that gave us a rate that was under $50 a month, for both of us. That's a number we could manage.

After about a month, or so, of us being enrolled in the market place health company, I received a rather surprising email. It was from the social security office, and since I'd been self-employed, or so I thought, for most of my life, I wasn't ever expecting to be involved with social security. I didn't think I qualified for any financial assistance. But that wasn't why they were emailing me.

They contacted me to let me know that I had been enrolled in Medicare part A since September, 2020. Medicare par A covers hospital stays for surgeries, and things of that nature. I was shocked to know that I had insurance for the last 8 months, and didn't know it. But again, that wasn't the gist of this particular email. They were sending me a bill for part B, that was scheduled to go into effect in July, 2021. Part B covers doctor's visits, labs etc.

I was miffed at receiving the bill, as I didn't enroll myself in Part B, and had decided to stay with the marketplace plan, so I decided to call the social security office to see what this was all about. Yes, I had Cancer. Yes, I was broke, but the government was about to step in to help me. I never, and I mean, never, expected the government to help me at all, so I started to do some research.

During the call, I was informed that the marketplace had given the social security people my information, and because of my age, 67, they had enrolled me. I had actually qualified for Medicare at 65, and if I had enrolled at that age, it would have been a little cheaper, about $20 a month. As a result, my premium was going to be about $160.00 a month. I didn't know how I was going to pay for that, so I decided to stay with the marketplace plan. That decision was made in April, 2021.

At the onset of July, when the Medicare part B bill was coming due, I decided to call the social security office again to fully see what my options were. I wanted to see if I had to enroll in Medicare, or could I just stay with the marketplace health plan. They said I could stay where I was, and that I could always enroll in Medicare down the road, although at a higher rate, as the longer you wait, the more expensive it gets.

I talked it over with my wife, and we decided to bite the bullet, and enroll me in Medicare part B, although that's more than we thought we could afford.

In order to meet the new expenditure, we got financially creative, and found ways to swing it. My health issues are not going anywhere, and I'm going to need to have good insurance, as a Colonoscopy is in my near future. I'll deal with that issue when this Prostate issue is over with, as that's for a future book…

In order to justify my new monthly bill, I assessed, and subsequently, reorganized my finances. The first thing I looked at, was my cable TV and internet spending. I was spending $180+ a month on those 2 services alone, and we didn't have any movie channels. So, I decided to "cut the cord," as they say, and happily waved goodbye to AT&T, or more accurately, Direct TV.

I also, looked into other non-essential spending's, and found fast food to be a large culprit. We have since limited our fast food and restaurant visits. You'd be amazed at how much that has saved us, and I'm sure it's better for us from a health stand point, as well. Win! Win!

With my monthly budget adjustment, and my marketplace health card now securely planted in my wallet, I made an appointment with a urologist. It was scheduled in 2 weeks.

Then, just prior to my Urologist's appointment, I decided to call social security again, just to make sure I was doing the right thing in staying with the health market plan. They said it was ok, but…and when I say but…I mean but!... That's when I was informed about this incredible stroke of financial fortune that was about to fall my way. The kind lady that I was talking too, said to me.

"Did you know that you have ten years of social security money waiting for you to claim?

"What!" I exclaimed. "How can that be? I've been self-employed my whole life."

"Evidently, 35 years ago you worked for a 10-year period, and paid into the system. You have equity built up that you can collect. It's fortunate you decided to wait until you were 67, because that lets you draw the maximum amount."

"Lucky I waited 'til I was 67? Hah" I laughed. "I didn't wait, I didn't know."

She went on to explain that I would be receiving a monthly stipend of around a $1000.00 a month, and out of that, since the social security office and Medicare are governed under one roof, social security would automatically pay my Medicare bills, and send me the balance. I was floored.

Armed with this stroke of luck, that quite frankly I had earned, I removed myself from the marketplace company, enrolled in Medicare part B, and went about my day.

Prayer

O Lord, keep me conscious of Your everyday presence, especially in these times of uncertainty. Empower my mind to accept the reality of Your presence. Lead me to accept the knowledge that You will never leave me, nor forsake me, and that in every doubt and fear in my life, your eyes are ever with me. Be glorified forever and ever, in Jesus' name.

Prostate Cancer Let's Talk!

Chapter 3 - The Urologist

"When you go through deep waters, I will be with you. When you go through rivers of difficulty, you will not drown. When you walk through the fire of oppression, you will not be burned up; the flames will not consume you"

- (Isa. 43: 2 - NLT)

Two weeks had passed, and the day to visit the Urologist had arrived. My wife, once again, kindly drove me to the doctor's office, and I fidgeted the whole way. Nervous would not best describe my feeling. Scared to death might be more accurate. I knew that this visit was going to be a bit different, and was definitely going to be a much more thorough exploration, shall we say.

At the hospital, we signed me in, and went to his office to wait the requisite amount of time for the doctor to arrive, about a half hour. Then, a tall, gray haired man in scrubs, and a covid/surgical mask walk in.

"Good morning," he said. "My name is Doctor Evans. Let's see what this chart has to say."

After perusing the chart for a minute, or so, he said.

"Ok, it says here that your prostate in slightly enlarged, and that your PSA level is an 8.3. Not terrible, but definitely something we have to look at. Let's get started."

His first directive was to send me to the bathroom to fill up a cup with pee. I naturally assumed that my urine was needed to get some read on what's in my system. That was a wrong assumption. When I got back, he laid me on the table face up, and proceeded to do a sonagram of my pelvic area. I nervously quipped. "Gee I hope it's not twins." He wasn't amused. I guess here's heard them all.

He showed me the sonagram, and informed me that I had left urine in my bladder. I saw a yellow dot on the sonagram that confirmed that. Evidently, not totally clearing your bladder is a symptom of trouble in the area, and he noted that.

I sat up, and he looked at me. Then, the words that I was dreading came from his mouth.

"Please lower your pants, bend over the table, and lean on your elbows, it's a more comfortable position."

I just froze, and readied myself, thinking, *"uh oh…here it comes…"*

I knew what was about to happen, as I am no virgin to this exam. Other than the fact that he spent significantly more time "exploring" the region than what had transpired on my first foray as a "bottom," excuse the pun, the exam was not painful, just annoying. Dinner and a movie might be appropriate, however.

"Well, you do have a growth, and it's covering the left side of your prostate. Surprisingly, your prostate seems almost normal in size, but the growth is of concern."

We talked for a while, as I fed him questions. After he felt that I had satisfied my curiosity, he told me what was to follow. He said that a biopsy, a procedure that would take samples from the growth to see if it was cancerous or not, was needed.

"Cancer!" I again, thought. *"Oh, shit! He too said the 'C' word!"*

"What's that going to entail?" I asked. Again, excuse the pun.

He told me that I would be put to sleep, and in a 15–20-minute procedure, samples would be taken from different areas of the Prostate, I would then, simply wake up, and be able to go home that day. I had never been put to sleep before, and the thought was terrifying.

We talked for a while longer, as I expressed all of my fears and concerns. He assured me that the procedure would go fine, and that I would not feel a thing. He also, told me that he was 70, although he didn't look it, and he had just gone through this same ordeal himself a few years prior. It made me feel at ease, knowing that we were of similar age, and that he could relate to my concerns and fears. Thankfully, I was at least comfortable with my doctor.

Ok, let's summarize... I've gone from ... "not a care in the world" ...to... "oh shit, I might have Cancer!" All, in about 6 weeks. Damn, life changes fast at this age.

Now, let me stop here and say, this book is not going to be maudlin in nature. If nothing else, this book is an adventure, hopefully with a happy ending. An adventure about facing the inevitable health situations we all are going to face at some point. Unless you get hit by a bus, at some point, your health will become an issue.

I am also, not down about this, so far, and let me stress, "so far", as I have not gone to my "next" appointed procedure. Currently, it's Sunday night, August 17th, the night before the biopsy, and on this night, I've decided to document my journey, and write this book.

In the morning, I'm scheduled for 2 scans, starting at 10:30 AM. These scans will reveal the extent of growths I have. Once deduced, there are 3 options I'm faced with.

1. It's just a growth, and not Cancer.

2. It's Cancer, but limited to the Prostate only.

3. It's Cancer, and has spread to either the Lymph Nodes, or to my bones.

Now, that's a scary thought, and this night's sleep will be a restless one.

Prayer

I now know, and confess today, that God's with me always. He is my ever-present help in times of need. He quiets my soul with His love, and keeps me safe and secure in His presence.

God is with me always, even to the end of this age. I will not let fear rule my heart, from this day forward. In Jesus' name...Amen

Chapter 5 – The Biopsy

"Fear not, for I am with you; be not dismayed, for I am your God; I will strengthen you, I will help you, I will uphold you with my righteous right hand." – (Isaiah 41:10)

Monday morning showed up, and after a very restless night, `my wife, lovingly enough, drove me to the hospital. We arrived about a half an hour before I was scheduled, and we sat quietly in the waiting room. Every possible scenario that I could ever imagine, flashed through my mind. The biggest concern was simply not waking the f*** up. Yup, I said it... "Not Waking The F*** Up!" I was terrified about that. This be my first surgery; I was crazy with fear. I hadn't slept but 3 hours the night before, and my lack of sleep, only added to my anxiety. I was simply having a hard time reconciling to myself, the fact that they do this every day, and it's a one in a zillion shot that I won't wake up, but that little zillionth was all I needed. I was scared to death.

When my time arrived for the biopsy procedure to take place, I was ushered into a waiting room where I was instructed to shed my clothes, put on this cute pair of yellow socks, and a johnny, a sort of paper gown with an open back. One must remember not to put this garment on backwards, it could be quite embarrassing, or maybe a proud moment for some…Not me, however.

I laid on the table in the pre-op room, and waited for about 45 minutes, all the while asking the attending nurses question after question about what I was about to experience. I'm sure I annoyed the hell out of the them, but again, this being my first time, and I, one of an inquisitive nature anyway, kept rifling off questions.

This incessant questioning followed me into the operating room, which had a classic look. Machines, big circular lights, a half a dozen masked people. You get the picture.

Once positioned in the middle of the room, they hooked me up to an IV that would deliver my sedative, then they rolled me onto my side.

I kept firing questions, and with having absolutely no awareness of me nodding off into la la land, I, simply woke up back in my room, groggy, but amazed that it was over. There was no counting backwards from one hundred, or anything like that. One minute I was in mid question, the next in my room. It was amazing how time had no meaning for me during my sleep. I was out for about 20 minutes, or so, yet it felt like a second, well actually, even shorter than that.

The doctor, still lurking from behind a mask like a thief, came in and informed me that the procedure, and by this point the word "procedure" was starting to irk me, had gone as planned. I was instructed to get dressed, and when I could go to the bathroom, (urinate) a precaution to make sure my bowels had returned to normal, I could go home.

That was it. I got up, got dressed, went to the bathroom, and walked out to my car with my wife, and she drove us home.

As you can see, so far, all is going well. The procedures, to date, have all been painless, and the staff has been extremely understanding of my fears, and as kind as could be.

The next act in this multi-part stage play, is to visit my Urologist to get the results of the biopsy. Is it Cancer? Is it localized? Has it spread? What are my treatment options?

Prayer

Heavenly Father, with my voice I reach out to you today that I believe Your Words and precious promises for my life and family. I believe that heaven and earth will pass away, but Your Words will never pass away.

O Lord, there are times I struggle with my faith, but Your Words are ever true. In Jesus' name – Amen

Chapter 6 – The Results

"I sought the LORD, and he answered me; he delivered me from all my fears."

(Psalm 34:4 NIV)

Another doctor's appointment was scheduled for late August, 2021. This was the consult where I was to be informed of the results of the biopsy. I was optimistic that I was Cancer free, feeling invincible, but unfortunately, optimism would give way to reality, as the results of the biopsy were not as favorable as I had hoped. The growth, which only sat on the left side of my prostate, was indeed Cancerous.

I was informed that I had several options, Chemotherapy, Radiation, Hormone therapy, or the removal of the Prostate using a procedure called, *robotic prostatectomy, a procedure using robotic arms.* But, before we could determine the right course of action for me, as each case is specific to each person, there was another step that needed to be performed… I would require full body scans…two of them. One for the bones, and one for the soft tissue.

These scans would help us decide the proper course of action, as they would reveal, in depth, the location of the Cancer, letting us know if the Cancer has spread, or is localized on the Prostate only. I was praying for localization, as the alternative, seemed more than I had bargained for.

He further explained that these scans aren't 100% accurate. There is always a chance that on the molecular, or cellular level, that one or two cells might drift off of the Prostate. That would be determined at a later date, but for now, these scans are step one in my fight against the 'C'.

Prayer

Father, deliver me from my present troubles and predicaments, for I declare that God is my Deliverer, and always

rescues me from every trouble, in Jesus' name. Amen

Chapter 7 - The Scans

"Now this is the confidence that we have in Him, that if we ask anything according to His will, He hears us. And if we know that He hears us, whatever we ask, we know that we have the petitions that we have asked of Him." – (1 John 5:14-15)

It is now scan day, August, 18th, 2021. I'm scheduled for one scan, the soft tissue scan, at 10:30 AM, the other scan, the bone scan, at 1 PM.

The first thing they did, at 10AM, was insert an IV. Then, they injected me with a radioactive die that's needed for my bone scan, which is scheduled for 1PM. The radioactive material takes several hours to fully penetrate the bones, so the bone scan was to be done later.

If you're reading this, and you must be, you'd probably like to know if this hurt…it did not hurt. Just a small prick as they inserted the IV needle, but, and trust me on this, as I am terrified of these things. It Did Not Hurt…A slight pinch, but I manned up…

After I received the radioactive fluids, which only took a couple of minutes, they walked me down the hall, and into a room, where center stage sat a large, white, circular device, a donut, about 2 feet thick, with a radius of about 3 feet. Extending from in front of that, was a long, thin, sheeted table. This device, or scanner, is used for soft tissue evaluation. This scan will reveal if my Cancer has spread to any surrounding soft tissue regions, like my lymph nodes, etc.

The attendant laid me down on the table. Then, using the IV insert, which was sticking out of my arm from the earlier use, he injected a saline solution. This was to clean the area, he said. This time, however, it hurt a bit, or rather stung. You know, like adding salt to a wound.

After that, he injected another scan fluid specific for this scan, and started the procedure. This was a 2, maybe, 3-minute procedure. You don't feel anything, or hear anything from the scanning device. You just lay there and wait for scan to be over, the IV to be removed, and to get the word to get up.

So far, everything was going smoothly, and we, my wife and I, had a couple of hours to wait while the radioactive die worked its way into my bones. We just made small talk. I fidgeted.

I did take this time, however, to do some praying. My relationship with God has been, well, a Godsend, especially during all of this strife, and has been a constant for all of my life.

I asked for relief from this bane, but also, gave thanks for my family, my close friends, and my extended families. Their support and prayers, have meant a lot to me. A veritable prayer army was organized on my behalf, and I couldn't be more blessed with their outpouring of love. As a Christian, a husband, a father, a loyal friend, not to mention, an ordained minister, I was taken aback by the shower of love extended to me. Thank you all very much. Continue your prayers, as we are not out of the woods yet, but I know your love is being heard, and will be answered.

Prayer

Father, I refuse to fear. When the need arises, and I am required to consult experts and professionals, I will do so, but I will not allow my mind to fear for any reason, for You have not given me the spirit of fear, but You have given me wisdom, and a sound mind. In Jesus' name – Amen

Chapter 8 - Scan 2 – Not Like The First.

"He that dwelleth in the secret place of the most High shall abide under the shadow of the Almighty." – (Psalm 91:1)

It's now 1PM, and for the second time today, they've come to take me away… Ominous sounding, I know. This scan is not like the first scan, which was a soft tissue scan, and took about 2 or 3 minutes. This second scan is a bone scan, and the due to the density of the bone, it requires a lot more time to complete, approximately 25 minutes. They are, once again, telling me that there will be no pain, that I won't even have a sense that a scan is being done, and that there won't be any loud noises, as in an MRI, just a steady flow of picture taking. I thought to myself, *"I'm good with that…"* Little did I know.

Now, I am of a thinking ilk, and I like to know exactly what to expect from all these procedures. Knowing what is coming really helps me get prepared. I can deal with pain…if I know it's coming. Surprising me is not in my wheelhouse.

Well, I asked the attendings what this scan would entail, and they told me that my arms would be strapped to my side, and feet bound. This was to prevent my arms from covering any other bones.

They asked if I was comfortable, and I responded.

"Ok, let's get this started."

The camera lens was slowly lowered towards my face, and stopped about a half an inch from my nose, blocking my vision from seeing anything but the cross hairs of this contraption.

They backed away, and told me not to speak, or move at all.

"Stay Still…" they ordered.

All I could think of was, *"I hope I don't get an itch from this Corona mask I'm wearing, that'll drive me crazy."*

About 5 minutes into this procedure, I started to get a touch of claustrophobia, a malady I've had since I was a kid. I'm simply not a fan of tight places. I instantly recalled the time, when on my wedding day, on the way to the Justice of the Peace office, the elevator stopped in between floors. My claustrophobia kicked in big time that day. I immediately thought it was a sign, and started to panic, but the elevator started moving, and my soon to be wife just laughed, but inside, I was terrified. All I wanted to do was get out of this moving crate. All she wanted was to do was get married.

I laid there rationalizing, that I'd have about 20 more minutes to endure this fear that was engulfing me, and I tried telling myself that all was ok, that I'm not going to die, that I'm not going to relent to this terror, but I couldn't do it, so, I semi-screamed to the attendants to stop the procedure.

"I need this to stop!" I shouted. "I need to take a break. I'm not sure I can do this."

They stopped the camera, and rolled it back so I could see the room, or more accurately, the ceiling. The attendants stood over me, and I explained to them that I tried my best to rationalize the situation, and control the fear, but I knew that I wasn't going to make it the full 20 minutes that I had left.

One of the nurses, in a reassuring manner said.

"We managed to get the pictures of your head, so you're good to go there. We can now move the camera down. You'll be able to at least see the ceiling, and won't feel so trapped."

"You know?" I said. "You could have told a guy that the camera would be moved systematically down my body, and it wouldn't stay positioned over my face for the duration. I probably could have made it to the end had I known this was to be done in stages."

They apologized for not telling me that little tidbit, even though up front, I was very specific about knowing how this would unfold. They repositioned the camera around my neck area, and we proceeded.

For the next 20 minutes, they would shoot a section, then stop, move the camera down, then shoot again. It took about 5 repositioning's of the camera to finish, and I had no further sense of angst. All went well.

After the shooting was over, they unstrapped my arms and legs, and I got up from the table and started to leave. But, before I could get to the door they asked if I was going to be around any babies, small children, or pregnant women over the next 24 hours. Surprised at the question, I said no, to which they replied that I'd be radioactive for the next 24 hours. I wasn't expecting that, and laughed.

"Gee!" I thought… *"Maybe I'll turn into the hulk…"*

All in all, this wasn't a bad experience. There wasn't any pain, and all I had to deal with was my personal phobia. I'm sure there are others that have this problem, and I mentioned it so you'll know that after about 5 minutes, you'll be good to go.

Finished with all that was to be done today, my wife drove me home, and I relaxed for the rest of the day. I just hoped and prayed that the results of these scans would be in my favor, and that my Cancer would be localized. Only God knows, but I'll be spending some quality time with Him this evening, dwelling in His secret place.

Prayer

Father, in Your presence is protection, guidance, and joy. This is where I long to dwell, And I know You will show me how to dwell in your presence, in Jesus name. Amen

Chapter 9 – The Surgeon's Consult

"I rise before dawn and cry for help; I wait for Your words"-
(Psalm 119:147)

This is the follow-up appointment at the hospital, to discuss my surgery. I had already made the decision to have the surgery to remove my Prostate, so the alternatives were not discussed.

You do have options at this point. Surgery, my choice, is not the only alternative. Chemotherapy, Radiation treatments, or hormone therapy, are also choices, but all of those would require weeks of daily visits to the hospital, and there would be some side effects that did not sound appealing to me. At my age, removal seemed the best, and most thorough option. I was good with this decision.

After waiting the requisite time in the outer office, surrounded by an infirmary of patience, we, my wife and I, were sent to a small waiting room. After a short time, a nurse came in. I was expecting the doctors who were to perform the surgery, but the surgical nurse was quite knowledgeable on what was to transpire, and I felt very comfortable with her. She answered all of my questions, and concerns.

After patiently letting me wade through my questions, it was her turn. I was a bit surprised when she informed me that they would require an MRI of my pelvic area to get a more in depth look at the Prostate area. I was a bit agitated that I wasn't told of this beforehand. Not so much because of the procedure, as I want them to have all of the information they can get, after, all, it is me they are invading, but the fact that I would need to make another trip to the hospital and spend a half day dealing with more tests, I wasn't happy.

They also, needed more blood work, which again, would require more time at the hospital. I wasn't expecting one more round of bloodletting…It is what it is.

I now, have a pretty good idea of what's about to happen over the next few weeks. After my MRI, which is in 5 days, they will schedule my surgery, and the ordeal will begin.

Armed with this new knowledge, I must admit, I'm a bit frightened. So much so, that sleeping has been a problem, and nightmares a constant. Recently, one such vivid dream saw me laying on the operating table, surrounded by a team of doctors. I remember screaming, as they cut me. I looked at the surgeon, who was holding a bloodied scalpel in his gloved hand, and he just shrugged his shoulders. I could see in his eyes he was, enjoying this. Then, a nurse who was standing next to him, chimed in.

"This might hurt a bit." She said. "Your insurance company only approved your surgery. However, they didn't approve your anesthesia. This will only take a minute. Just try to relax."

I woke up in a sweat, rolled over, and spooned my wife. One never really knows the comfort of a loved one until you get scared out of your wits. I am blessed to have her in my life.

Speaking of my life, I thought it prudent, at this juncture, to address my daily life outside of my doctors' visits. I would be remiss if I didn't let you know how I was dealing with the other side of me.

As of today, the day before my MRI, I just flew in from El Paso where I played a wedding gig. Yes, I am a musician, as well as other things, and these activities have not waned just because I've been 'diagnosed.'

I've just finished a 6-month run of every Saturday night playing wedding gigs, in which I flew all over the country. I saw some cool places, but the ending of this tour couldn't have come at a better time. I am tired, and need the time ahead to beat this Cancer, and continue on with my life. I do have other job-related responsibilities, and will continue with them up until the day of my surgery. I'll then set aside some time to get back to full strength. Any surgery takes its toll, and this is no different.

This unexpected diagnosis has put me in a good frame of mind as it relates to my health, however. I have since, started eating better, and I've lost some weight. I plan to adopt a healthier lifestyle, since this peek at my possible future sees me riding out my life sore, and out of shape…not pretty.

When these things happen, one must find a positive spin. Strengthening my faith in God is on the top of the list. Followed by making sure that my family knows how much I care and appreciate their love and attention. Then, finally, getting into better shape. I want to finish this thing called life, gracefully, and although I may have to deal with other health concerns later on, I'd like to be able to meet those challenges in the best shape I can be in. This will give me a better chance at beating whatever I'm to face. My family deserves to have a husband and a dad in their lives for as long as possible. I will try to do my part in that joint effort.

This book, as stated earlier, is not a doom and gloom look into my ordeal with Cancer, however. I'm hoping that the words written inside these pages can help someone, even if it's only one person, in dealing with this, or any type of health malady one may face.

There are ways to stay positive, and aide the bodies healing process. Dwelling on the negative, is not healthy. All that blackness can severely retard your body's ability to fight off undesirables. So, find something you like to do, and do it a lot. Be happy for whatever time you have left, as every day is a blessing. So, stay blessed for as long as you can.

Ok, back to the matter at hand. After my MRI, I've opted to have the robotic surgery, as this is the least invasive surgery available today, September, 2021. I give the date in case this is being read 50 years in the future. How optimistic about the sale of this book am I. I'm laughing, as I'm typing this, but you never know when something will hit the public's collective nerve. Stranger things have happened. I'm not writing this for sales, however, although that would be nice, but my experience in dealing with this Cancer is worth putting to paper, so, I'll trudge on.

The tests will be evaluated, and I'll be scheduled for my surgery. From what I've gathered, so far, this is what I'm to expect.

With this robotic surgery, there will be no large incisions, as in the scalpel days. There will only be three small cuts, two slits about two inches in length, on either side of my stomach, and a small puncture in my naval. That's not too much cutting, considering they are taking out an organ.

The surgery entails the removal of my Prostate, and while they are there, they might be taking out my Lymph Nodes. Again, another surprise, as this was the first, I was hearing of this. I was told that they are not needed, and could possibly house a small amount of Cancer. This was not a big deal, as getting rid of all this shit inside me, is of paramount importance. I don't want to go through this a second time, just because they weren't thorough enough the first time.

After the removal of my troubled areas, and before they close me up, they will insert a catheter into my penis that will extend from my bladder to a receptacle, a bag. This will help me expel urine during my recovery period. I was told, that recovery from the need to use the catheter would only take about a week to ten days, then they could remove the catheter. I could then resume normal urinary function. I've been told by several people, who have been through this, that it's really not that big of a deal, ... *'It sounds worse than it actually is'*, is what I took from their assessments. I'll give you the skinny from my perspective when I go through it.

In the meantime, I'll get the MRI over with, give them some more of my blood, and be back when the results of those tests are in. With that new information, they'll schedule my surgery.

Prayer

__Lord, from now onwards, whenever I find myself in any trouble, or in dealing with any malady, O God, show me the way of escape. May these prayers voiced with the knowledge of Your presence, be answered, in the name of Jesus Christ. Amen__

Chapter 10 – The MRI Experience – Well, I Tried

*"Nevertheless, I will bring health and healing to it; I will heal my people and will let them enjoy abundant peace and security." **(Jeremiah 33:6)***

Well, my MRI "was" scheduled for this morning, September 1st, 2021, and I stress "was," because this did not go as expected. I simply couldn't handle it.

I have, what I thought, was a touch of claustrophobia, well, I was wrong. After this experience, I may start using a harsher word than 'touch," to describe my phobia, but however decide to label it, it came and reared its ugly head this morning.

I stated earlier that this fear had previously attacked me during the bone scan, but I got through that once they moved the plate from my face. Also, I was not totally enclosed for that scan. The camera on the bone scan is only about 2 feet by 3 feet and it's only placed on top of you, not all around you. You are never fully enclosed. as with the MRI machine. I thought I could readily handle the MRI. I was sooooo wrong.

When I first walked into the dungeon, and I call it that because it was dimly lit, and had an evil overtone to it. I'm sure it was my over reactive imagination, but it had Sci-fi written all over it. I quickly tossed that ominous feeling out of my head, and tried to ready myself.

In the middle of the room, sat the beast, a huge, and I mean huge, circular shaped ring with a platform extending from its ominous mouth. I knew this wasn't going to involve any pain, so I was good to go, or so I thought.

They asked me to lay on the platform, so they could slide me in for a test run to see how I would react to the cramped conditions. I asked the attendants if would be able to at least see the ceiling, and they said I could. This made feel a little more comfortable, and I thought, *'piece of cake, I can handle this'*… Man, was I ever wrong?

What I hadn't expected was the fact that they were about to slide me in, then raise me up. At this point, I was literally encapsuled in this thing so tightly, that after only 30 seconds of my 'test' period, I was already asking to be taken out. I was so crammed into that tube, I simply started to panic.

Let me stop here, and try to explain what this 'panic' feels like. It comes on slowly at first, then gradually accelerates until I start feeling a little cramped. The cramped feeling continues until I'm no longer simply feeling cramped, I start to feel trapped. Once, I'm to the trapped stage, and to the point where I feel that I can't get out, I'm in a full panic. If I let it get to that point, I'd be screaming, kicking, and flailing my arms in an attempt to get the hell out of the tube by any means possible. IV's would go flying, and I'd be trying to shimmy myself out of the bottom, into the open area.

Now, I've never gotten to the point of feeling fully trapped in any previous bouts with this panic, but I know how it would turn out if I ever got there. It would turn out just as I've described it, not a pretty, or glamourous sight by any account.

I shook those thoughts out of my head, as they slid me out of this white cocoon, and I sat up to discuss this problem. I knew I needed this MRI before they could schedule a surgery date, and I didn't want to delay this any longer, but I knew, that all of the intellectual rationalization I could muster, was not going to beat this panic. I knew this scan, on this day, wasn't going to happen, so I asked about alternatives.

They, the attendants, whom I must stop to recognize, have all been extremely nice, understanding, and knowledgeable of all that I've been going through. Thank you JPS, Fort Worth, for proving me, and the community, with a staff that really cares. That starts at the top, so kudos to all.

They informed me that about 40% of their patience experience some degree of claustrophobia, and that I shouldn't feel bad. I laughed at that prospect thinking, *'You can throw 'feeling bad' out the window,'* I was really pissed, and downright angry with myself for being such a baby.

She, the nurse, went on to say, that they do have other methods of scanning, an open MRI, but they were expensive, and not available in all hospitals. This could cause a problem for me, so I asked about any other alternatives. I know this didn't happen, but I swear I saw a wry smile peek out from behind her mask, and a glint in her eyes when she said, *"...there's always, Xanax!"*

I have never taken any drugs of this sort in my whole life, so I had to ask what was involved with that drug. She said, that I wouldn't care about anything once the Xanax kicked. They could drop a house on me, and I wouldn't flinch. She went on to say, that almost to a person, the Xanax worked in eradicating any sort of panic, and that I would sail through the MRI scan unaffected.

I have my doubts, but my wife and daughter swear, that I simply won't give a shit about the scan, or anything else for that matter... I guess I won't be driving home that day.

Prayer

Heavenly Father, today, I declare that You will satisfy me, and my household with a full, healthy, and long life. And in the end, we will receive His salvation. In the name of Jesus Christ. Amen

Chapter 11 – The MRI – Round 2

"The LORD ***is my strength and my defense; he has become my salvation. He is my God, and I will praise him, my father's God, and I will exalt him."***

(Exodus 15:2 NIV)

It's Thursday, September, 9th, 2021, and I just got back home from my 2nd MRI, and I'm pleased o say, no, I'm actually proud to announce, that I've made it through the MRI unscathed. All of my pre-surgery tests are now finished, and I'm ready to get this operation thing over with. I'm not looking forward to that day, but in two weeks I'll be living on this planet without a Prostate. Maybe

I'll lose some weight from having one less organ to carry around, that would be nice.

Speaking of weight. Since this all started, I've dropped roughly 15 pounds over the last 4 weeks. Not a drastic loss, but a sustainable pace for me. I've simply changed a few eating habits, like eating more veggies, broccoli, green beans, etc, and more fruit, mainly blueberries, strawberries, and melons, cantaloupe, and honey dew. I've also, started eating a small breakfast, a meal that I've routinely skipped for years, as for me…coffee "is" breakfast.

My breakfast consists mainly of instant oatmeal with milk. (2% - If you haven't switched to 2% yet, you should. After a few weeks you won't taste the difference, and whole milk will feel like cream to you.)

In preparing the oatmeal mixture, in a bowl I add, 1 oatmeal packet, milk, (approx. 1/3 cup) and some blueberries, then microwave the mixture for about a minute, and voila! …breakfast is served.

This easy breakfast provides much needed fiber from the oats, essential nutrients from the berries, and calcium and vitamin D from the milk. I've always liked oatmeal, but hadn't eaten it in years. This little change is a very healthy way to start my day.

For lunch, I've been eating the melons. They fill me up, provide some mid-day energy, and are low in calories. That's all I need for lunch.

As far as protein is concerned, at dinner time I've been eating baked chicken. I haven't graduated to fish yet, and I absolutely love shrimp, so I can see those items being a nice change from chicken, but at this point, chicken hasn't gotten boring yet. I'll drop some of my recipes here, so you can see how I prepare some of these things. I'm a closet chef, and I love to cook, and maybe some of these recipes will work for you. I don't like to labor over food preparation, so these meals are fast, and not labor intensive. I like to get in and get out so that I can eat. I do use a lot of spices however, as I like heat, but, not so hot that you can't taste the food. To me, heat without flavor is a waste of good food, and money.

I usually add some vegies to my dinner meal, and on occasion,

I've managed to have a few vegan days, mainly because I didn't feel like cooking, and surprisingly, I didn't miss the meat at all. There have been times in my life that I've toyed with the idea of going vegan, but, somehow that lifestyle change doesn't seem to be a sustainable option for me. I don't need to eat red meat to any degree, mind you, and for now, chicken is a satiable option…at least for now.

Well, let's get back to the day at hand. I had a 7AM MRI scheduled, so my day started early. I had trouble sleeping, as the angst of sliding into that tube again had me tossing and turning all night long. That damned claustrophobia is a real deal bear, and I was dreading having to give this another go, but my over active imagination was thankfully interrupted as the alarm went off at 5:30AM.

I got up, showered, grabbed some coffee, a bowl of oatmeal, and sat in front of the TV watching Sports Center, while my wife got dressed. I'm very lucky to have her in my life. I know the divorce rate is high, but I can be honest and say that to have my best friend, and ardent supporter of all things me, metaphorically holding my hand throughout my life for the last 37 years, at the time of this writing, well, that's truly been a blessing from God.

After arriving at the hospital, and going through the usual sign-in procedures, it wasn't long before I got the call. They ushered me into a small waiting room where I was administered an IV into the back my hand. This would be used later to inject dye into me, which would take place in the last 5 minutes of the MRI. The MRI itself, would take roughly a half an hour. Much too long if you ask me.

When I walked into the room where the beast resided, the huge donut shaped machine with the platform extending from it, beckoned me. Having been through this before, I was terrified, but earlier I had taken a prescribed drug, Atazan, and although I didn't feel like it was working, I had a stare down with said beast. I was told to take it about a half an hour before I arrived, and that should be a sufficient amount of time for it to get into my system, well they lied. I felt nothing.

Scared, and a bit fidgety, the attendant, who was a different person than the first time, was extremely helpful in keeping me calm. He knew that I had already tried this once before, and the claustrophobic bug had bitten me badly. He too, had been there before, not only as an attendant, but as a patient. This fear of enclosed spaces, is not unique to me. They told me that roughly 40% of people they give the MRI to, have at least some touches of this fear. That didn't make me feel any better, but at least I knew I wasn't alone in this war.

The attendant looked at me and asked. "You Ready?"

"I guess so." I said. "However, I don't feel like the anxiety meds are working yet. I've never taken anything like this before, and I was expecting to feel something."

"They are." He said. "They aren't like drugs that make you high, or anything like that. They just curb your anxiety. You're not in the machine yet, so you don't think they are working, but you're awful talkative, so they must be doing something."

I just thought to myself... *'hell, I'm always talkative...'*

He asked again if I was ready, and I responded with a nod. Then he stopped, and asked me a remarkable question.

"You know, I can put you in feet first, if you think that will help?"

"What!" I exclaimed. "You can do that? That wasn't even an option on my first foray with this thing. They just shoved me in, motored the platform in, and raised me up until I couldn't see anything but the beast, and it was almost touching my nose. I didn't last 30 seconds before I knew that I wasn't going to last the full 30 minutes, so I stopped the procedure before it even got started. But feet first, sure, let's give that a try."

"You'll still be almost all the way in, but you'll be able to at least see some of the ceiling, and you'll be out in the room. Do want to give that a shot?"

"Hell, yes!" I optimistically exclaimed.

With that, he put me on the table, motored me in up to my neck, then raised the platform. I was still cramped, as my arms, which were folded across my chest, were crammed against the walls of the demonized donut, but I could at least see, and having my head out into the room, seemed to keep me from freaking out.

Now, I don't know if the drugs were working, or the fact that I was in this thing facing out had helped, but I did know that I was going to be able to get this done. I also knew, that I had to get this done, or they would have to postpone my up coming surgery. My life is sorta dependent on getting this cancer out of me, so I manned up, and told him to get this show on the road.

Just before he left the room, he asked what kind of music I wanted to listen to. I told him Smooth Jazz would be fine. That's when he punished me. He played Kenny G for a half an hour straight. I don't know how much you know about Kenny G., but he popularized the circular breathing technique that sax players use. They breath in through their noses, then out into the sax mouthpiece, creating a continuous flow of air. When mastered, they can play a note indefinitely. Well, I got one note for almost half of the time I was encapsuled. Now, that's punishment.

The procedure itself is painless, but the noise, or racket that the machine itself makes, is surprisingly loud. It's real loud in fact. So loud that the music, which was turned up pretty loud to begin with, almost disappeared in the din, save for that one dreaded note that Kenny was playing. That note cut through everything. It was mind numbingly offensive.

Well, I managed to get through the MRI unscathed, and after getting dressed, I went out to meet my wife in the waiting room.

My wife, ever the talkative one, and unbeknownst to me, had told everyone in the waiting room of my fear of this machine, and that I had taken the Atzan only a half an hour before I went into get the MRI. Several people, who were waiting for procedures, and had been through this before, told her that an hour at least would be needed for the Atazan to kick in. I wasn't privy to this information until I was later told, and I was a little surprised that the gathering in the waiting room gave me a round of applause, as they realized I had "made it.". I laughed, boughed, then exited.

"What was that all about?" I asked my wife.

"Nothing," she said. "Just the usual smattering of approval given to someone who had weathered a storm. It's all good. Plus, it's not the first time you've been applauded for something."

With that behind me, we headed to the labs where I was scheduled to give blood and a urine sample. After my donations, we left the hospital, and I drove home, as I wasn't feeling any effects from the Atzan. I'm glad that's over with. But I'm proud I got through it.

Prayer

Lord, I live within the shadow of My Heavenly Father, sheltered by the Holy Spirit. God alone is my refuge, my place of safety; He is my God, and I am trusting him completely. In Jesus' name - Amen

Chapter 12 - The MRI Results

"Do not worry about your life, what you will eat or drink; or about your body, what you will wear. ... Who of you by worrying can add a single hour to his life" (Matthew 6:25-27)

The results of this MRI was different than what I had expected. Some good news, some bad. First, they said that it looked like my Cancer was just on the left side of the Prostate, which was a good thing. But my Prostate had enlarged a bit, and it was touching my bladder on the right side. Fortunately, no Cancer was creeping into the bladder from what they could see. All in all, they felt like the Cancer was isolated, and they should be able to get it all out. We'll see when they actually go in there, but for now, I'm staying optimistic.

One of the other things they mentioned took me aback. They said that on a scale of 1 to 5, in the risk of returning department, I was a five. Since my brother had Prostate Cancer, although 15 years ago, the simple fact that he had it, put me in the high-risk category. High risk in the sense that it had about a 30% chance of it returning. I'll go every 3 months for a PSA test, for a year, and if my PSA readings are 0, then I'll be ok. There is no guarantee that Cancer won't come back, but if I can get through a year with a score of 0, I'll be happy.

With all of that, they scheduled my surgery for 2 weeks into the future, September 24th. Before I could do that, however, I needed to get a Covid test, which was no big deal, and proved negative, and have an obligatory pre-op consult. This took place over the phone.

The consult was a simple one. They asked a bunch of questions, like was I allergic to any type of drugs, or had I ever had previous problems with anesthesia. I answered no.

They also, told me of my night before routine. I was not to eat or drink after midnight, and at 6PM, I was to drink a Calcium Citrate liquid that would have me in the bathroom all night. This was all standard, as cleaning me out just seemed prudent. I had instructions on washing as well. They gave me an antibacterial soap, that I was to use 3 times before surgery. Morning before, night before, and the morning of.

I followed all of the instructions, and headed to bed. My surgery was 5:30 in the morning, so I'm sure sleep won't exactly be what I'll be doing, and it wasn't. I tossed and turned all night in angst of the morning's doings.

Prayer

Lord, take every form of sickness away, and cause Your healing, blessings, and peace to be with me and my family. Let the Blood of Jesus Christ flush out every kind of virus, bacteria, and disease out of our bodies. In Jesus' name, I pray.

Chapter 13 - The Surgery

"Have I not commanded you? Be strong and courageous. Do not be frightened, and do not be dismayed, for the Lord your God is with you wherever you go." (Joshua 1:9)

So, here it is. Friday morning at 4AM...D Day, or more appropriately... 'C' Day, and I'm taking my last antibacterial shower. I didn't sleep well last night, as this next 10 hours has been haunting me. I don't know what to expect, as I've never dealt with surgery before. Sure, the biopsy saw me being put to sleep, but they say this time will be a bit different. The biopsy, although I was out, was more of a local. This time, I'll be all the way out. Whatever that means.

The first thing they did, was have me get undressed, and then they slid into the johnny. With my butt hanging out, I crawled onto the bed, got as comfortable as I could, and prayed I would get through this. They started 2 IV's, one in each wrist. By this time, I've had a few IV's, and I'm getting used to them, so at this point, I'm just flinching a little, as they stick the needles into the back of my hands. They do a lot of sticking needles in you, as they are constantly giving you stuff, and constantly taking blood as well.

I need to stop for a moment, and take the time to mention the staff and surgeons that performed this operation on me. I was at JPS Hospital in Ft Worth TX., and these people are amazing. The surgeon, Dr. Hutcheson, and his staff, came in prior to the surgery, and they all took time to talk to me, answer my questions, and give me a rundown of what was about to transpire. From there, I met the Anesthesia people, and then, the nurses who were going to be involved.

I must mention the nurse that got me prepped for the surgery. Her name is Marjorie, that's all I know, but she was an angle in keeping me calm, and she patiently answered all of the questions that I was rifling at her. She is truly a special person, as was everyone. Nurses, Elaine, Rosette, and Jessica, were especially helpful in keeping me sane, both in pre-op and post-op/recovery.

Ok, back to the surgery. At admitting, they asked if I wanted my wife to get text messages during the surgery, and I checked yes. If you are going to do this, have them text your spouse, or person who is there with you. It is nice for them to stay informed. My wife was told that the surgery was to be about 2 hours long. Mine took 5 and a half hours. She was getting messaged every hour, and she said it surely helped her stay calm. After the third hour however, she was starting to get nervous, afraid that something had gone wrong. The texts help her stave off her anxiety.

My surgery, did take an inordinate amount of time, as my Prostate had swollen, and was leaning up against my bladder. The robots, which are used in this of type of surgery, had to make several extra incisions that were small, and one rather large one, in order to work their way into position to remove my Prostate.

All in all, it took 5 and a half hours, and the doctors said that it was a difficult surgery, but they managed to remove my Prostate, and the adjacent lymph nodes, without disturbing the bladder. That was a blessing, and a testament to the skill of my surgeons.

Finally, back in my room, as I certainly had no recall on the actual surgery, I started the awakening process, which took a while, as I had a lot of Anesthesia to wade through, but after a half an hour, I was getting coherent enough to talk to my wife.

It's an amazing thing when they put you out. You don't remember nodding off. One second, you're asking questions, then you are simply wake up in your room. It's quite an experience.

Once totally aware of my surroundings, I woke up to find a catheter extending from my penis, which was being used to empty urine into a rather large plastic bag. It didn't hurt, but it was disconcerting. I'd never had a tube coming out of my penis before, and it's rather alarming the moment you see it.

I spent the rest of the night just resting, and watching some TV with my wife, as nurses paraded in every 2 hours to give me pain meds, or take blood. The blood work was to check if I was getting any infections, which fortunately, I wasn't.

My wife, Dawn, spent the night with me, and she woke up the next morning in more pain than I was in. Sleeping on the chair next to me, was not a fun night for her, but thank God she was here though. I don't know how I could have handled all of this on my own. I'm glad I didn't have to.

The next day, I was released in the late afternoon, about 3:30PM, as one night was all that was needed to make sure that all went well. Not too bad, all things considered.

Before I was discharged, the doctors came in to tell me what they had found, and it was as good of news as one can expect. They said it looked like they got all the Cancer, and that my bladder, although leaning against my Prostate, showed no signs of Cancer. I was relieved at their findings.

The only real instructions they gave me was to return in 8 days to have the catheter removed. Once removed, I would be wearing an adult diaper for about a month or so, as I would not have control of my urine output for a while. I was told of this beforehand, so it didn't surprise me, and I took it in stride.

The last thing they left me with was that I had to return in 3 months to get a PSA test. If it shows a reading of zero, I will be Cancer free. I'll still have to go back every 3 months for a year, to get a PSA test, but that's just a blood test, and not an inconvenience, as opposed to needing Radiation, or Chemo. Those two treatments are administered weekly, and for a long time. Thank God, at least at this juncture, I won't be needing any of those procedures.

In wrapping up this ordeal up, as I'm now 5 days removed from my surgery, I'm still dealing with the catheter, but only for 3 more days, then they will remove it. The removal will require them to deflate a balloon that's holding the catheter in place inside the bladder, then pull it out. I've been told that it's not a painful procedure, that you'll only feel the thing slide out, and although that will feel weird, all in all, it's not painful.

I have to thank God for the blessings involved here, as being ushered to the doctors by my wife and daughter, Amber, for a visit, were truly a God send. I probably would have waited much longer to get a checkup, and who knows what that might have wrought.

When I get the results of my first, in the series of PSA tests that await me this year, I fully expect to be Cancer free. If you are going through this, may your results, as well as my results, be as positive as possible. I'll be praying for you.

In closing…God has seen me through this, and with my love for Him, and my family, I fully plan to enjoy what time I have left. Hopefully I'll see 90 something, and hopefully you will too. God Bless!

Thoughts From The Author

Thank you for taking this trek with me. I hope, that in some small way, I have given you a glimpse into what to expect if you ever face this all-too-common ailment. The sheer number of men over 60 that will deal with some sort of Prostate issues are staggering. All I can say is, that they say I'm Cancer free, for now, and I feel blessed.

Get tested, stay positive, and bring God into your life. It always helps to have someone watching over you.

God bless you all….Edgar Lloyd.

About The Author

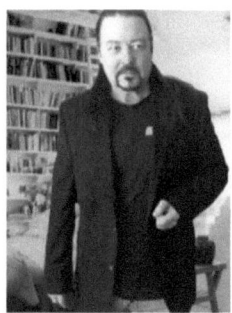

Edgar Lloyd...Minister, Author, Narrator, Composer

Born outside of Boston, he spent his formative years splitting time between Massachusetts, and Baltimore, where at an early age, he showed excellence in athletics, music, and creative writing. His athletic prowess, as a running back, earned him a full scholarship to Colgate University, where he studied music, literature, and theoretical science.

After attending Colgate, he toured the country as a performing musician for several years, before settling in the Dallas/Ft Worth area, where he's continued his career as a composer, performer, author, narrator, husband, father, and ordained minister

He authors, sci-fi adventures, historical fantasies, religious books, and educational books relating to the music, audio, and voice over professions.

Other Book Available –

Books 1 & 2 from the series "Adum's Kronicles" featuring Christian Super heroes – the "Triumvirate"

Assimilation Book 1

https://www.amazon.com/dp/B0178KOCXU

Shatter – Book 2 -
https://www.amazon.com/gp/product/B07TRNY8X5/ref=dbs_a_d ef_rwt_hsch_vapi_tkin_p1_i0

Web page for more info - https://audioartcafe.com/edgar-lloyd-narration%2Fvo

www.ingramcontent.com/pod-product-compliance
Lightning Source LLC
Chambersburg PA
CBHW031925240526
45464CB00022B/999